LIVING THE SEASONS
of Life
FALL AND WINTER

LIVING THE SEASONS
of Life
FALL AND WINTER

How to Relate to, Assist and Enjoy
Your Aging Loved Ones

BY MARILYN LAHR

XULON PRESS

Xulon Press
2301 Lucien Way #415
Maitland, FL 32751
407.339.4217
www.xulonpress.com

www.LivingTheSeasonsOfLife.com

Printed in the United States of America.

ISBN-13: 9781545622261

THANK YOU!

Thank you for purchasing this book. I'd be truly grateful if you'd take a few minutes to REVIEW this book and give your feedback on Amazon and on my website. Your feedback is always welcome and appreciated and may help others decide if this is a book that may be of interest to them.

If you would like to know of future books or stay in touch with articles I am writing, please go to my website at www.LivingTheSeasonsOfLife.com

To contact Marilyn:
Website: www.livingtheseasonsoflife.com
Facebook: www.facebook.com/ livingtheseasonsoflife

Email: livingtheseasonsoflife@gmail.com or email Marilyn from her website

By mail: Marilyn Lahr
PO Box 773852
4545 SW 60th Ave
Ocala, FL 34474

DEDICATION

I WOULD LIKE TO DEDICATE THIS BOOK to Elizabeth Gail Robinson, who by the way she lived her life, showed many what it means to be a "friend". I am honored to say she was my dearest friend. Without her love and belief in me I may have never written this book or all the ones to come.

She lived the true meaning of friendship and held a space of unconditional love. She encouraged my growth, my belief in myself, and reminded me so often that the trials of my own life were an opportunity for growth in compassion for others.

For 22 years she held my hand and my heart through the good times and the tough times. My hope is that this book will help others through those times as well.

She left this earth plane a short time ago but I believe with all my heart she now cheers me on and celebrates with us from "higher ground". Together we will celebrate with you as you hold a space of love and create times of joy with those you love and care for.

Marilyn

ACKNOWLEDGEMENTS

I WANT TO ACKNOWLEDGE:

Monte Taylor who led the way for me as an author and has been an inspiration and example of one who is intellectually brilliant but speaks from the heart. Monte spent many hours helping me get started, and most of all I want to thank him for his devoted friendship. Don't miss his book on Amazon, *The Power of Heart Language*. The information in this book, when applied, can improve every area of our lives.

Gail Robinson for all her unending patience, love, encouragement and input.

My devoted friends, and especially Tina Myers, for her friendship and untold hours of listening and giving me feedback. I couldn't have done this without you Tina.

My wonderful children who love and support me, have given me beautiful grandchildren, and who listen to me at times when I know it is difficult to do so, but stay by my side and bring the joy to me that every mother longs for. Together we are living the principles of this book as I have lived them with my own mother. God bless you.

I would also like to acknowledge all the beautiful seniors who have shared their memories, their lives, and their hearts with me. I have learned from you and I love you.

Marilyn

TABLE OF CONTENTS

PREFACE AND DEDICATION

MANY YEARS AGO, AS I WATCHED WITH love and concern the aging process of my mother and Aunt Gladys, and was doing programs in retirement homes, I started writing a book I would one day publish called, *Living the Seasons of Life – Fall and Winter*

I shared some of my writings with my Aunt Gladys one of the last times I saw her, and tears streamed down her cheeks as she said to me, "You have captured what we experience as older people, and no one seems to understand. You are a voice for those of us who have no voice. Please share this Marilyn, maybe someone will listen and understand!"

That day is finally here and so I dedicate this book to my own dear mother Clarissa Mae Lahr and my dear loving Aunt Gladys who were the light and love in my life and shared with me the most beautiful love one could ever hope to know. God shone through both of them and if anyone wanted a demonstration of what love really is, they gave it; and I was privileged to live in their love.

And, to my brother, Ron Lahr, who taught me how to laugh and whose laughter I miss. Ron gave me memories that I cherish and it is a blessing to carry that laughter with me through the Fall and now the early Winter of my own life. I have every reason to believe if I live to be 100 and beyond I will still find laughter in the memories we shared. What a gift! Thank you, Ron. I hope I can bring some joy into the lives of my readers as Ron did for me. *Prayer, laughter, and getting out in nature, are God's greatest healing agents and we need them more than ever at this point in life.*

And so in memory of my mom, Aunt Gladys, Ron, and the scores of beautiful seniors who have shared their lives with me, I share this with you and hope there are those who will be listening. *It is my desire that this information will greatly assist those who are perhaps searching for answers on how to meet the needs of their aging loved ones and how to best relate to them. It is also for those loved ones who need you to understand the 'winter' of their lives.*

You see, the greatest pain the elderly go through is not just loss of the use of their bodies or minds but the loss of dignity, much of which could be avoided *if* their families and those who care for them would take the time to understand.

My intention in writing this book is:

- 1st   To be a voice for the elderly
- 2nd   To help those who love the elderly to know how to better understand and relate to them.

- 3rd   To bring out many understandings and ideas that will give great relief to those who have no voice or are afraid to say what they really want and need and to help their families and caregivers to know how to make these last years or moments of their lives as loving and joyous as possible.

This book comes in three parts:

PART 1–"Is Anyone Listening?" … To what I fear, I want, and I need.

With each stage of life our wants and needs change. No one has prepared us for growing old, and the lives of those around us are so busy we are afraid to ask. Often it seems no one wants to listen but we don't deserve to be set aside, our needs marginalized by those we have given birth to and/or loved and assisted to get where they are in life. So let's have an open discussion about what those who now depend on us need us to hear.

PART 2- "The Heart Cries"… of those who have lost their voice.

This section may be a bit difficult to hear but to not do so is to leave your loved ones forever feeling they are not understood and, if ignored, it can leave you with a lifetime of regret.

At a certain point of the aging process the most loving parent or loved one may feel they shouldn't tell you what they are really going through – they don't want to be a burden. They are often frightened and feel they have no one to tell, *or* they may actually, mentally or physically, lose their ability to communicate and are, without your understanding, locked in "solitary confinement" without a way to tell you what they are going through.

First, let me say if this happens and they begin to live in an alternate reality that is happy, although it may seem to you a childish fantasy, *do not* criticize them or try to bring them back to a reality they can no longer bear. If they have found a happy place, be it ever so childish or unreal, let them be happy. It is their mind and bodies way of coping with their current reality.

But sometimes their world just becomes a world of silence, and yet there are things they want you to know. This part will be sharing with you their inner thoughts and story. Knowing this, if you understand it, you can make it much easier for them and for yourself.

**PART 3–"Creating Beautiful Memories" …
with your loved ones that will last a lifetime
and beyond.**

This section of the book will be giving you an endless wealth of ideas on how to create and preserve wonderful and meaningful memories with your loved ones. There is no reason you have to sit and say nothing to one another, or try to tell them things and have to repeat over and over or try to correct them, or feel you have nothing to do or say. *I will share with you ideas that I have seen work like a miracle to bring the sparkle back in their eyes, to fill them with joy and gratitude; and you as well. This will be the fun part and will create for you and for them beautiful memories to last a lifetime and beyond!!*

A note on how to receive the most benefit from this book.

Think of this as a workbook which you will reference again and again over time. As such, I encourage you to highlight memorable passages and make your own notes throughout the margins and in the back of the book. Perhaps list out your own thoughts as a new idea comes to you.

Also, as the years go by and your loved one ages, different parts of this book will become more relevant. So, I encourage you to periodically re-read the book to pick up again on the information and ideas that now apply to your situation.

I hope you will not read it quickly or only once and think you have absorbed its value. Many of the statements, suggestions, and observations are ones that need your most sincere pondering and consideration. Asking yourself if this applies to your situation, and if there is anything you want to change in this particular area, is the way to the greatest benefit.

(You will find some blank pages for your notes in the back of the book.)

INTRODUCTION

FALL HAS ALWAYS BEEN MY FAVORITE season of the year. I've often said, "It brings out the gypsy in my soul!" I want to run with the wind, have a new adventure, play in the beautiful colored leaves, take in nature's beauty and be a part of it. So, I found it very strange about 14 years ago when I was in my early 60s that fall brought upon me a strange nostalgia and at least a mild depression. What was this about?

As I looked out into the beautiful colored leaves on the sugar maples outside my window and pondered this strange feeling, the voice in my head said, "It is fall in your life Marilyn – not just outside your window. It is your reality!" Until then I didn't fully realize I wasn't still 30 years old with all of life before me. The next thought was, "Oh good Lord, if that is true.... I'm facing winter! The winter of my life!"

Please understand this book is written for all ages and seasons of life. For those who so very much want and need to be understood and for those who need to understand. Know that just as the seasons follow each other, so do the seasons of life. I hope this book will give voice to help us understand that; both for others and ourselves. It seems no one has really prepared us for the changes of seasons.

Each stage of life is never fully understood by those who have not yet experienced it but in order to have some level of understanding with each other and relate, we need to try, and it is to that end that I share these words with you.

I have now experienced all these seasons except the one that is coming near and that one I have experienced through my own mother and dear aunt and all those wonderful people who have shared with me in the retirement homes.

You see, elderly people do in some ways experience feeling like a child again in that they reach a point where they must have others look out for them. This is much harder than being a child because we have known what it was like to be self-sufficient, so we need a great measure of your understanding. It is very hard to accept regressing instead of progressing. To accept you can't do some of the things you once did. To have to wait for someone to help you do the things you were once able to do for yourself.

And…if those around you don't 'get' that, it makes it worse by a hundredfold because that truly does add insult to injury. This is the time when you must reach deep inside yourself for a level of respect, patience, and understanding in order to not make us feel worse or rob us of what dignity we have left.

We may not have a lot of time left to create some last beautiful memories together, so rather than avoiding that topic or pretending it's not so, let's face it full on and, with understanding, make our time together as wonderful as possible.

It is my desire to create greater understanding by being as honest as I can. *Some of these words you may find upsetting but denial is not going to help us make the most of our time together, however, with understanding there are many things that can and will be shared here to help us navigate these, until now, uncharted waters together with love, joy, and many more great memories.*

CHAPTER ONE

Part 1: Is Anyone Listening – to my wants and needs?

I WANT TO SPEAK TO YOU, THE FAMILY member or caregiver now about the fears, wants and needs of your loved ones. I speak sometimes in the first person as I am one who is entering the early winter of my life and I am living through the beginning stages of having to have these conversations with my own family. And, I am keenly aware of the conversations that may be coming, having lived through it with my own loved ones and being friends with many others in this season of life.

I also understand, and want to help your aging loved one understand, that their part in this is to do their own inner work and to do and be as much for themselves as they can.

Entering the Winter of Life

In early winter you may be telling yourself, "I'm as good as I ever was – maybe better." If you are one of the fortunate ones that may be true, but somewhere in the winter season of life things begin to happen that may be alarming both to the family and caregivers, and very much so to the one who has entered winter. It can be extremely uncomfortable to talk about the changes that are taking place but it is imperative that we do so. This is not the time for silence or to pretend it isn't happening. There are real changes to deal with and that takes perhaps the most open and honest discussions you and your loved ones have ever had, and the most courage. This book is written to help you with that.

In this section I want to share with you the fears of loved ones who now need help to maintain their quality of life.

First, I would like to share a few thoughts with those who need your care. You may want to let them read this part for themselves.

(**A few words to those of you who have entered the "winter" of life and may be needing help from your loved ones**.) This book is being written to help those who have become your caregivers to understand a great deal of what you are going through in this transition of your life where you may not be able to completely take care of yourself. I will be very clear and direct with them about the fears, needs and wants of those of us who are losing some of our abilities. But… I do need to address a few thoughts with you, the aging loved one.

Your part in this will be to do the very best you can to understand their fears and concerns too. Just like I never bought into the idea that because women are hormonal every month it gives them the right to mistreat those around them, age is also not a license to be abusive in any way to those who are doing their best to help. This is difficult for them too. Nor should we, who are needing help, be too sensitive to the point of denying the changes and our need for help.

I know this is hard for you but the best way to navigate the changes you are experiencing is to recognize that they are creating changes in the lives of those who care for you too. Good open, honest, and loving communication is the only way through these changes. It might help you a great deal to read what I am about to share with your caregivers and I hope it will give you the ability to communicate openly with them – if only to point to a page and say "Yes that is how I feel," or, "That is what I want or need."

Be appreciative of all they are trying to do. *No one has all the answers for this transition without good communication on the part of all of you*. Don't be afraid to state what you are going through but do it as lovingly as you can and it will be much easier for all concerned.

(Now to those of you who will care for us.)

Our fears:

Losing abilities of mind and body. We all have moments when we forget names or simple things and sometimes we wonder if we are getting forgetful, but often in today's world it is just a sign of an overcrowded mind, so don't be too quick to assume the worst. Perhaps it's a signal we need to get out in nature and unwind a bit. It is, however, quite different when we see a pattern of not being able to remember what we did yesterday or we see the look on someone's face that lets us know we already told them this – perhaps several times.

What follows next can be traumatic if the other person responds with a sharp "You already told me that mom – several times!" Ouch – we feel scolded like a child, fear, and a sharp pain at your insensitivity. Often we have to push back both tears and anger.

It doesn't help us when you tell us that. Your sharpness or impatience hurts and the reality of your words frightens us. If you notice we are slipping, be gentle, kind and begin to look for some solutions. There are many "natural" products out now that are known to help with memory and, of course, there are medications; but don't be quick to give us medicine if there is perhaps a natural answer. There are many things that our bodies used to produce that decline as we age and some of these can be replaced with natural supplements and/or even change of diet. Be aware that we may not be eating right as we get too tired to prepare balanced meals.

You might want to do a "google search" first and ask for natural products that help with memory. Be sure and try those first as they have no side effects like drugs do.

Know that anything you are noticing about changes in your loved ones they may well be aware of and any reprimanding tone from you only makes the problem worse and more frightening to them. *It's your turn to calm us and keep us safe as we once did for you.*

It is also very disturbing if your loved one has led an active life and finds their ability to do the things they used to diminishing. Be very aware of the need to encourage us to be more active before it's too late, but don't scold or criticize. Those won't help but they diminish our self- worth and can send your loved one into a depression. You may need to insist a little to get us to do physical activities when we don't feel like it, but any activity is apt to lift our mood and build our strength. So try to think of something that might be fun – perhaps some activity your loved one used to enjoy. Maybe there is something you can do with us – a walk, a yoga class, get us to go to a balance class or a senior's dance. Or if you really want to see our lights turn on, take us someplace with you to see some beautiful things, or how about taking Mom out for dinner and dancing?

Don't be quick to write us off – there are probably many things that can be done. I'll talk about many more ideas in the 3ʳᵈ part of this book.

Another fear...Being underestimated by our children and others. *If you don't want us to get old before our time, stop underestimating us!!*

This one can be the worst!

Don't just assume our advice is outdated, our opinion not relevant, or that we can't do it, because of our age. This is a matter of respect, so stop and think before you brush us and our possibilities aside.

The rolling of your eyes or your attitude cuts like a knife. Because we are older doesn't mean we don't have anything to offer or are incompetent. In fact, the opposite may well be true.

In other countries there is respect for white hair. They know with age often comes wisdom. I'll give you this much …. I truly believe as a friend of mine once said, "When you get older, if you have learned from life, you become an elder with much to offer. If you have not learned from life or have become embittered by it, you've become just another old fart." But give us the benefit of the doubt as there may be a head and heart full of wisdom under those gray hairs. Give us a chance to offer our advice or show you what we can still do.

There has never been a time in our lives when we need you to believe in us more. We have enough doubts about ourselves as the things that once made us feel valuable are fading and faltering. Your belief in us, your putting value in our opinion means the world to us. Give us every chance to show you our value by asking our opinion, by listening when we speak and by letting us make our own decisions when possible, and let us help in some way.

Another big fear... Losing our right to make our own decisions

Part of understanding what our aging loved ones are going through is the ability to put yourselves in their place, for in another decade or two you may be exactly where they are now. Think how it must feel to someone who has lived through what they have lived through. Done all that they have done, including raising you, to not be allowed or considered in making the choices that now affect their lives!

They truly may not be able to make the best choices for themselves but they should be allowed to try and to have their input and choices very carefully considered and if at all possible, honored. *Their dignity and their will to live may depend on it.*

Closely connected to this is our fear of being marginalized when we share our ideas or, just being overlooked

Don't be in a hurry to think our opinions aren't important or practical or are unneeded. Boy, do we feel that. Just be aware of how sensitized we may have become about feeling that our input is not considered or valued.

Fear of Being a Burden

The most common comment I hear from the elderly is… "I don't want to be a burden to my family." We have lived our lives to create greater opportunities, ease, and possibilities for your life and to think that now we might become a burden is an unbearable thought, both because of its potential effect on you and, to have to admit to ourselves that we can't take care of ourselves any more. It can cause depression and even self-loathing.

It is very unfortunate that our society does not teach, as other cultures do, that your parents will do the best for you that they can and one day you will have the opportunity to return the favor. If indeed you can get your head around that, that this is your opportunity to do your best for them, it will make all the difference in the world in the emotional messages they receive from you!

Which leads to our next fear....

Fear of Feeling Impatience from our Family or Caregivers

Nothing is worse than doing our very best, yet feeling our very best tries your patience with us, frustrates you, and affirms our worst fear... that we indeed are a burden and you are disgusted with the burden.

I emphasize "feeling" because as we get older our gut catches what our mind may not. We "feel" it when you are anxious or irritated with us. It is conveyed in your energy, your eyes and your touch.

I remember my days as a massage therapist. The most important part of my training was when my instructor said, "Don't touch someone when you are in a bad head space. They will feel it." So, I determined to always allow myself time before giving a massage to get myself centered and in a peaceful place inside myself, knowing that I had no right to pass on my concerns or frustration to someone who needed a healing touch.

So giving massage became very therapeutic for me as I calmed myself no matter what was going on. It was a discipline but certainly had its reward. *Your loved one may now be the angel on assignment to teach you to slow down, calm yourself, to not carry with you and pass on to others the angst of your day.*

A thought you may need to ponder. You may feel like this is requiring a lot of you and that very likely will be true, but at what point when your parents were raising you did they say, "That's it! I won't do any more for you. I've done enough! I don't care about what you want or what you think you need." Even sometimes when looking back you know they went way beyond their comfort zone to give and do for you? When did they stop doing anything they could for you to make you happy or your life better? Now it is your turn. Just as they were your only source of protection and provision, you may now be their only hope of being cared for in the way they need and/or deserve.

Fear of Death

Many books have been written on this topic so I will only touch on it here. The best way I know of to deal with the fear of death is to talk about it. Not talking about it doesn't make it go away and, believe it or not, some of the greatest peace you and your loved one can know is to discuss it freely and completely. Your loved one knows when it is coming near and when they must think about it alone, they feel they must face it alone. Don't deny them the tremendous relief, and even joy, the two of you can share as you talk about this openly and lovingly together. And from your standpoint you will find the loss of their physical presence much less painful if you have shed your tears together about how you will miss the physical presence of each other. Tremendous bonding and peace can come from talking this through. Check with hospice workers for advice on this. The whole hospice program is built around making the 'transition' as easy and peaceful as possible.

This entire book is written to help you live to the fullest now and be at peace when that time comes because you and they know you've both done all you can to enjoy each other now and to prepare for the end of your physical journey together. And… a part of that is the next fear.

And another very great fear…fear of leaving unsaid things that should be said and understood between us.

Perhaps it shouldn't be so but it is very true that many family members have a hard time saying the things to each other that they really want or need to say. Sometimes these burn like a fire within us because we want our feelings and thoughts to be known and understood. These fall into many different categories both for you and for them, such as…..

- Unexpressed feelings of love
- Sometimes unresolved hurt or anger

- A story of a part of life that we've wanted or needed to share
- A hope to be understood in some area
- Unexpressed longings

Whatever they might be, sometimes even a word can make a difference in a life, more than can be imagined. Those who remain have to live with those unspoken words, and/or questions for the rest of their lives – either the words they longed to hear from their loved ones or the ones they wanted to express and never can now that their loved one is gone. And sometimes what was left unexpressed could have painted a very different picture in your mind or theirs by hearing "the rest of the story" or unraveling a misunderstanding, and that resolution can give us relief and closeness. Or, worst case, and it's really not that bad, we can agree to disagree, but love anyway.

Garth Brooks sang a song with a haunting question... "If Tomorrow Never Comes…..??" You fill in the blanks and see if there is something you need to talk about today, now, that could make a difference for you or for them. You may need to be the one to start the sharing by expressing anything unsaid on your part. Take it slow and don't try to force them or expect an immediate response. Let them absorb what you have said and they will share when they are ready. Your words, and their feelings, may need to sink into their hearts for a while. The end hope is always that it will bring more love and understanding and bring down those unspoken barriers between loved ones.

And, kindle warmth and peace within your hearts and relationship.

My father died at the young age of 59. I was a daddy's girl and loved my father dearly. I was on vacation with my family when he passed and there were no cell phones then. My mother told me that dad, who almost never placed a phone call, tried to call me at least 3 times in the last two days before he died. We later found out dad might have had reason to know he was dying. He died suddenly of a heart attack. He never told anyone else what it was he wanted to say or ask me. I have wondered about that for 38 years now. Don't let that happen to you if it can be avoided. Don't put it off. And be sure to encourage your loved ones to say to you whatever is in their heart.

AND, if you have strong feelings of love, express them every time you have a chance!!! "I love you" can be the most healing three words in this world. If you want to give your loved one good medicine let them know and hear it now and every chance you get. What are the words you want your loved one to hear when they lie their head on their pillow at night? Or just when they think of you? Getting older can be a very lonely time, and just knowing they are loved makes them feel less alone and as if you were holding them in an embrace.

Our Wants and Needs

These two will overlap a good bit but bear repeating. ***Please don't just read the heading and think you*** *know what it says*. Read the content, that's where the real meaning and understanding comes.

Our wants:

To not be overlooked

There is something that happens when our children are grown and out on their own that is difficult to explain unless you've been there. For 18+ years a good parent's life revolves to a very large degree around the raising of our children. We delight in it, we create relationships with other parents and our children's friends. We join organizations having to do with our children's activities. To a very large degree our identity comes from all of this, and then, if we have done a good job of parenting, our children leave home.

We are no longer needed for our advice or assistance as we have been for a couple of decades or more. All of that is understandable, at least mentally, though not so much emotionally, but then a next phase comes where our kids' lives get so busy we are often "overlooked". We sometimes actually feel *"invisible"* – not needed and sometimes not wanted. This can be a cause for depression and often is. It may be real or imagined but it "feels" real to those whose days may be filled with little except thinking about family and days gone by. Living perhaps only on memories and needing some new ones.

Bottom line – we still want to be wanted and needed in your lives. That is the next point.

Our want is to know we are still needed in your lives. Every time you ask our opinion on something we feel needed. Or if you ask us to help you with something, large or small, your requests make us know we still have a place in your lives.

One of our greatest needs…to be listened to

While the fullness of your lives is expanding, ours are getting smaller, and even if we have made lives of our own your opinions, phone calls, visits and every way you show you care, as a general rule, mean more to us than all our friends combined. And we need you to listen to us. That need grows as we age and even if we have told you the same things many times – feeling we are heard by those we love means more than almost anything or anyone else.

I won't belabor the next two points but please give them consideration.

To be wanted – We sometimes feel like we are last on your busy list, so a word or two lets us know we are still wanted and an action on your part to include us goes a very long way.

To be appreciated–I'll just say that if there is anything you enjoy or appreciate about us be sure and let us know. Being appreciated is a very important part of feeling loved and valued.

Our needs:

To be a part of things – Include us in all that you can. Your lives are busy and full – ours often are quite empty unless you include us.

To have companionship – our friendship circles get smaller as we age; both because we can't get together with friends as often as we used to and because we may have lost many of our friends to old age. Especially if we have lost our mate we very much need companionship in any way that you can help make it available to us. Your companionship always being the most important.

To have meaning. If we have any interests or hobbies, you showing interest in them gives us meaning. If you take interest in what we say it gives us meaning, and if you want to be with us or talk with us, or if you ask our advice – it gives us meaning.

To be touched. When my mother reached a point where she could no longer speak and later when she didn't remember who I was, touch would momentarily bring her back. I learned that holding her hand, or holding her or even spooning with her when she was lying down brought some kind of awareness. She would stroke my arm or smile and seem to "come back" with physical touch. I do believe touching helps people to not slip away to another place if we do it often enough before that time comes – it could delay our loved one slipping away from us.

To know we still make a difference. This has already been said in other ways but if there is anything about our time together that makes a positive difference for you, let us know. That keeps us present with you. Perhaps ask us to say the blessing or share a parting prayer.

To still have adventures... Oh my yes! Taking us for a ride in the fall, taking us with you on any outing, perhaps giving us a new experience of any kind brings us back to life. If we still live in our homes, come and spend a day or two or more with us and do some things together. Perhaps take us on a vacation with you for a few days.

To be able to tell our stories and have them appreciated. What a marvelous difference it would make if families made a habit of asking the elderly to tell their stories about family, memories, their childhood, our grandparents, travels they have made and so much more – and let the grandchildren know this is a special time and they will learn a bit of their history and they will learn about us and be able to pass that information on to their children. *Invite* us to share and make it special! Ask us about our favorite things. I'll do a section on that in part 3 of this book. Don't miss it!

To ask our advice because you know we have learned from life. What do you know is something your loved one took pride in about their life, their work, their hobbies, about health or their spiritual beliefs? *Few things mean as much to us as to know you still think our advice is valuable.*

To be given every opportunity to still express ourselves. Perhaps to cook something for our family, have you in our home, have you take an interest in our pets, flowers, our interests. To share a talent we have with you and/or our grandchildren. Perhaps support us in a new hobby.

We need you to teach our grandchildren to respect us and to take an interest in what they can learn from us. Teach them to ask us questions such as:

Some questions you and your children can ask....
What life was like when....

>*What life was like when you were a child, grandma, grandpa?

>*When you got your first TV? Is it true there were only 2 channels?

>*What was it like when there were no computers or calculators?

>*When you grew your own food. Did you? What did you grow?

>*How much was your allowance? How did you like to spend it?

>*The first time you met someone from another country. What country? Tell me more....

>*Did you go on vacations? Where? What were they like?

*What you were like when you were my age. What did you like to do? Were you shy? Who was your best friend?

*What are some of your best memories of Christmas as a child.

*Did you have pets? Ask us to tell you about them.

*Perhaps ask us to teach you how to bake a pie or sew.

(There is another list of questions in the activities section that follows.)

Let us have memories with you and our grandchildren *on our terms* and not expect us to entertain them but to share with them. Maybe teach them a song from our childhood or the top 5 tips about life that we would like to share with them. Encourage your loved one to share the lessons and wisdom they have gained from life. That reminds them of their value and the value of their lives – thoughts and feelings that will linger after you leave them.

In summary: Understanding these needs, wants, and fears can and will make all the difference in laying a foundation for the way you and your children and grandchildren will relate with your aging loved ones for the rest of their lives. Realizing what a frightening time this part of life can be for them will give you a different perspective and create loving bonds instead of divisions. Keeping things positive on your visits but having these types of conversations and activities will change the way you relate to each other, and when you go, it will leave Mom or Dad with a smile on their face – and I'm guessing one on yours as well.

My prayer is that you will read and reread what is here until it becomes a part of your awareness. Refer back to this information again and again and I promise it will dramatically change your life and the lives of those who love and need you. By the time you read Part 3 of this book you will be able to turn stress into joy. Read on....

CHAPTER TWO

Part 2: Heart Cries

THIS PART OF THE BOOK WILL BE BRIEF but is a collection of three of what I call "The Heart Cries" of those who may not be able to say these things to you, either because your loved one feels they can't or shouldn't say them or because they have lost the ability to speak, but these thoughts are locked inside them. I hope you will be very aware that when they reach the point they can no longer express themselves with words they are ever more keenly tuned into "feelings" – yours and their own. They read your face, they feel your energy. Don't think they don't understand or feel because they do, and often more deeply than ever. The elderly with whom I have shared these writings weep because by my sharing them they feel someone understands – they wish you did. (These are representative of some of the things that might be spoken from their heart)

You Think I Don't Understand

You think I don't understand how busy you are and how difficult it is for you to find time for me in your life. I do understand and I am proud of all the things you are doing with your life, for your children and your work, and I feel badly to add another burden to it. Do you understand you are all I have that matters to me in this life now and I don't want to be a burden but rather be love and joy in your life? I want that more than anything else but there is so little I can do. I often can't even use my words any more. I just feel it in my heart.

You think I don't understand what you feel when you are repulsed when you look at me now all skinny and sometimes unable to even feed myself, but I understand. I see it in your eyes. You are afraid of your own feelings and feel guilty because you may want to run or just stay away. It doesn't take words – I feel what you feel, but inside this old shell of a body still lurks a heart that longs to be loved and touched and to let you know how one smile from you is like someone just turned on the light in my darkness – one touch is like someone wrapped a warm blanket around my cold frail body.

Maybe I am a mirror confronting you with your own mortality. I can't tell you to not be repulsed or afraid but I can tell you every effort you make to be with me is appreciated more than you could ever imagine, and one day everything you have done to comfort me will comfort you. In the quiet of the night when you think of me you will know that you made me feel loved.

A few comments about if or when they must leave their home.

The most difficult decision you and your loved ones will make is when they can no longer stay in their home. If it is at all possible for you to make a way for them to live with you or another loved one please consider it because removing them from every-thing familiar can put them on a fast downhill slope. If that is not possible please be aware that the way they respond to you at the suggestion of leaving their home is coming from their tremendous fear of letting go of what is familiar. Please read on to gain some understanding of the thoughts and feelings they may be dealing with. If you can understand, as opposed to trying to convince them of their need to give up their home, it will make it so much easier on both you and them if they know you understand their concerns and their feelings as you help them make the transition. *(When the heart and feelings are involved sometimes the facts don't seem to matter, but knowing they are understood can make a huge difference.)*

Where Is My Home?

Why do I have to leave the place that holds all my memories at a time when my memories are all I have and many of those are fading?

Where is the rocker where I held my babies and sang them lullabies? My home where papa's slippers were still tucked under the bed – the last reminder I had of him each night at the end of long lonely days and I slip into bed. The home where I baked cookies with you, where we celebrated birthdays and Christmases.

Yes, I know times are changing but that is all the more reason I want to hang onto those things that are familiar to me.

The rooms of my home hold memories like movies I replay again and again. The walls hold the laughter and tears of our lifetime together. I can still hear your laughter as a child. I've left some of your little finger-prints on the walls and they make me smile.

I have been separated from all those dear to me – many have passed, including papa, and you children have moved on. I have only my home and my flowers in the yard, the tree I look out into every morning. The plants I have tended with care all these years. The birds that sing outside my window, little Chippy, my chipmunk friend whose antics make me laugh. Do you know how these comfort me?

How will I survive in a place that is just brick and mortar with no meaning to me? A place that holds no memories. I will surely be more alone than ever with only the faces of strangers around me.

You say you will come and visit and bring the children and we will create new memories – but will you really? Your life is busy and you will know I am "taken care of" so will you come? Will we laugh together, spend time together in this new place and make new memories? And what will happen to my things that mean so much to me? Will I forget more because nothing is familiar? Do I have any say in this or have I been stripped of the dignity of having a say in my own life?

I'm not trying to be difficult. I am frightened, more frightened than I have ever been in my life and I don't know if anyone is truly listening to me!

I need to know you hear me and that you care enough to try to understand. That you will give me my own choices as long as possible. And when and if it must happen that I leave my home that you will listen and honor my requests. I ask that each of you, my children, come and spend some time with me in this new place and create some memories. I ask that I can select things that will come with me to this "new home" – my rocking chair, my bed, grandpa's slippers, my family pictures, my mother's favorite teacup, papa's pipe. I ask you to let me make choices as much as possible.

And I will need to see that I am not forgotten. Include me in things that you do whenever possible. Come to my place and bring the children and teach your children to listen to and respect the 'story times' we have together so that I might have an opportunity for them to know me and remember the family stories I tell.

My heart aches now more than you can imagine and I will need much love and assurance from you when I must make this transition. When you are young you make many transitions and you make them with a great deal of ease because you know you have all of your choices ahead of you. I fear the choices I have left are few to none. I hope you are listening because I never thought this day would come for me and one day it will come for you. I hope when that day comes those who love you will be listening.

A Light in Her Eyes

This particular writing is a bit of a segue into the next phase of our journey together in this book as we find ways to bring life back into those who have slipped into a place where even remembering may be painful as they think these times are gone away and they will have no more. We will talk about many ways to make your loved ones have something to look forward to, and you as well.

A Light in Her Eyes

Several years ago I was doing weekly presentations/performances in retirement homes. My performances were designed to "engage", not just entertain. It was in lovely facilities and people were well cared for, and older couples were able to have their little apartment together and stay together.

I had decided to do this particular one in the dining room to have more space as I took them back in their minds to the old Grange Hall Dances.

I wore a square dance dress with full petticoats and began setting up my music. Lunch hour was over and everyone was gone except for one old couple sitting off to themselves. I watched as I was setting up and saw that she kept her head down all the time but with a word from him would lift it just enough so he could put a spoon of food in her mouth. I went over and spoke with the gentleman for a moment to let him know what I was doing and to please not let my presence make him feel uncomfortable or rush him in any way. I suggested he might like the music I was about to play. He nodded and thanked me.

I put on some fast fiddle music as the others gathered at the other side of the dining room and I began to dance to it. They were soon clapping to the music and tapping their toes. Seeing their response I got more and more into it – I loved watching them "light up". On one of my spins around the floor, I saw that the elderly lady who had been bent over the whole time I was setting up had lifted her head. I danced my way across the floor toward her and her husband and I saw a light come into her eyes and she smiled at me. Oh my, what a delight. I gave her my best performance and the smile continued. They stayed for the whole program and when I was finished the gentleman nodded for me to come over. He simply said, with tears in his eyes, "Thank you so much, I can't remember the last time I saw her smile." Oh my! Could anything be more rewarding?!

The whole purpose for my programs each week was not to just entertain them but to engage them, to help them "remember", to help them get in touch with the joy inside themselves. What a joy it was as they remembered "Their Favorite Things", shared their beautiful stories and told me that things came back to mind that they never would have thought of again....

One man's memory of delivering milk with his father in glass bottles and an old horse and buggy. Another gentleman over 100 years old recounting his story of a trip to Alaska in perhaps his 20s or 30s and how he reached a point and someone told him that Russia was a brief boat trip away so he paid a gentleman to let him use his boat and made his way across the waters and got out and stood on the shore and waved his arms in the air shouting, "I'm standing in the Soviet Union". He quickly left and made his escape back to the good ole U.S.A. And then one dear lady shared her memories of going to her grandmother's house when she was a girl where the highlight was her grandfather would bring out an old feather mattress and put it on the old iron bedstead in the yard and she would sleep out under a canopy of stars. I will not forget the sparkle in her eyes as she remembered a time filled with youth and youthful wonder and family.

What a joy it was to see a smile on a face that hadn't known one for so long!

And by the way, the 100-year-old gentleman danced a few steps with me just to know he still could sweep a "young lady" around the floor again.

CHAPTER THREE

PART 3: Activities for Enjoyment for Both You and Your Loved Ones

Creating Beautiful Memories
With Your Loved Ones
And…. Having Fun Doing So

THERE ARE MANY WAYS TO DO THIS AND I will give you a list of ideas and possibilities, some are simple things that may only take a few minutes while others such as my first five examples below are ways you can spend an hour or a day together having fun and creating memories that will warm your loved one's heart for a long time to come. (You will find lists and songs in the addendum.)

I will begin with a few of my favorites.

1st…**My Favorite Things**

We all remember the song from the sound of music, "My Favorite Things" – a delightful and joyful song of the simple things of life that bring a smile to our faces and bring delightful memories. "Raindrops on roses and whiskers on kittens…snowflakes that lay on my nose and eyelashes….." (When using this with your loved one you may want to bring some "props" a few pictures of the old days or pictures of things mentioned in the song. And get the CD or download the song off the internet. Then you have both audio (the music) and visual (your props) helping to wake up their minds and senses.

I decided this would be a wonderful thing to share with the elderly by first finding out what some of their favorite things were. I played the CD with the song and they sang along. Then I had a sheet of questions for them that you will find at the end of this book. Don't just give the list to them, you keep it and perhaps write down some of their responses. Then take your time and ask them one question at a time and really listen to and enjoy their answers.

This is a simple way to begin to "light up" their memory and their mood. For you to show an interest in knowing their favorite color, food, movies, song, and as you go further, to get into questions like…."What is one of your favorite memories of…your mother, your father? Your favorite childhood birthday? The place where you grew up? Your grandparents? Christmas, as a child, as an adult. Favorite vacation. Favorite pet. Their first love. Their first kiss. First dance. It's endless. Obviously avoid questions you know could be painful. Then listen, really listen, *enter their world with them as perhaps you never have before.* Hear stories you may have never heard and see the delight in their eyes as they remember things long forgotten but, remembering now brings delight. They will feel so loved and they will love you so much for taking them, in memory, to those places. In doing this you will feel a special bond between you. (*If you know some of the stories and characters they mention and they don't get them right, that's not important, don't break into the state of joy they are feeling as they are telling their story. Facts don't matter – the feeling does.*)

This can be continued from one visit to the next. There's no hurry, as you both will enjoy the answers. Keep the sheet you have written the answers on and when you get home, write down notes of things they shared that you may want to remember. This list will also give you ideas on what and how you can please them with pictures, food, adventures together, indeed "their favorite things" and it will mean a great deal to them to know you really listened as you bring some little token on a return visit. (Don't assume men wouldn't like this one. I have shared it with several and they do – very much.)

2nd...Favorite Idea: **VIRTUAL TRAVEL TO PLACES THEY HAVE BEEN or PLACES THEY WOULD LOVE TO GO**

This can be done in several ways, such as...

Ask them either where is the favorite place they have been or where is someplace they always wanted to go and didn't. Ask them what they would like to see and do in those places or what they remember of places they have been. (This is just to help you prepare for a future visit when you will go there with them from the comfort of their couch.)

Then begin to have some fun and plan a time when you will "go there together" so to speak.

You can begin by gathering pictures, perhaps a travel video, information, music, foods. Such as:

A trip to Italy....

> *You can perhaps pick up a tablecloth (plastic is fine perhaps with grapes on it, or white linen and crystal glasses if you prefer).

> *Gather pictures from magazines or ask a travel agent for some brochures.

> *Get a CD of Dean Martin singing those classic old songs for background music and/or use the music to spark a mood or activity such as dance. I've enjoyed dancing with partners up to 101 years of age, men or women.

> *Pick up some wine or sparkling grape drink and some cheese, or if you have the time and energy make a lasagna or get one from the freezer at the grocery store.

> *Perhaps you can get a couple of cute hats from Walmart for each of you.

> *Whatever helps create the atmosphere.

You can do this over and over again with different countries and places. Take them to Ireland – lots of fun music for that one. Take them to the islands and beaches of the world. Don't miss Hawaii – and be sure to give them a lei for that one along with a Pina Colada and some great music, a colorful scarf or a pareo – try the hula for some laughs.

Or, as I shared with you above, I once bought a CD called *"Fiddle Magic"* – you may be able to find it online – dressed up in a square dance outfit and reminded them of the old Grange Hall dances, did my best to tap my toes to the music and move around the floor. You should see the light in their eyes. Ask them about their memories of same or if they ever wanted to go to one. OR... get some music from the 40's, 50's, or 60's – their era, and invite them to the prom and create that atmosphere, and ask them if they went to prom. Ask them to tell you about their memories of their prom. (Perhaps buy Mom a corsage & come dressed up a bit).

Remember what it is you are doing, and that is to "turn their lights on" – to awaken good memories in their mind. You will see it in their eyes and it is so very rewarding. You can "bring them alive", spark their memories. Laugh together as you clink your glasses. Let them know you care enough to put the effort into having some fun. I promise you once you break the ice with this it will change your visits forever and leave both of you with warm memories.

Remember to snap a few pictures of everything you do with them and print them out and put them in an album or create a "Shutterfly" book online they can keep on their coffee table and share with others or look through when they are lonely and it will remind them they are thought of and loved!

3rd …Give them **A KID'S CHRISTMAS.** The elderly love being taken back in time and feel younger when you take them there. They often enjoy being a little playful too. In all of these scenarios it can really help if you dress the part – for instance… When I do a kid's Christmas I pull my hair back in two little pony-tails and tie them with ribbons. I put on a pink fleece long nightgown with snowflakes and I come carrying a sack (blanket) full of stuffed animals and I have a big lollipop or candy cane. I get a little silly with them by singing *I'm Gettin' Nuttin' for Christmas* and *All I Want for Christmas is my Two Front Tee*f get them to sing *Rudolf* with you and put on a red nose if you have one. Then begin sharing memories of Christmas, first theirs, then some of yours. Share some cookies and milk or tea and after an hour or so of sharing and you can perhaps sing along with a few of the sweet old classics like *White Christmas* or *Silent Night*. This doesn't have to be on Christmas, just anytime around the holiday. Bring the family and ask them to join in if possible. Letting them *remember* by being playful will bring that sparkle in their eyes you are looking for and a joy will linger in your heart and theirs long after you say goodnight or Merry Christmas.

4th ⋯ Have a **"HIGH TEA"** Take them back in time to when women wore pretty dresses and hats and had time to have tea with each other. I like to sprinkle rose petals on the table and use real china cups. I bake some simple cookies they might remember – like shortbread made with real butter – tastes they don't get in a retire-ment home. You can tell them ahead of time to wear a pretty dress. You can bring them a pretty hat (you can purchase these inexpensively at Wal-Mart if you like). Play some music from their era – perhaps something upbeat like *"Getting to Know You"* and use this time to get them to share some of their memories of a genteel time. Use pretty napkins and your best manners.

5th ⋯ Take them on **AN OLD-FASHIONED PICNIC** If you have or can buy or borrow a wicker picnic basket those are the best to set the mood, but a small cooler will do if you prefer. A red and white checkered tablecloth and napkins add a special touch. Your picnic can be in the backyard or go to a special park or a place they might like to revisit. My mom loved to go down by a little lake where she could feed the geese and swans (no longer allowed now). Use your imagination. You can prepare some of their favorite foods or just make it sloppy joes or sandwiches, potato salad and a piece of apple pie. Spread that pretty tablecloth and spend some time watching nature and reminiscing about days gone by.

Let's not forget Dad. While some version of all of these can be adapted to the aging gentlemen as well as the ladies it's good to remember that Dad would love to watch a football game with you or any other favorite sport while sharing a pizza and a beer or coke. Take him to a sports bar once in a while if he likes, or just plan ahead for an upcoming game on TV, your place or his. There is ten times the pleasure in watching sports activities with someone else, hollering, cheering or even placing a small wager.

A List of Ideas for Activities with Your Loved Ones

For me, the goal in creating activities with seniors is not to "entertain" them so much as to "engage" them, wake up their minds, turn on the lights. This creates much more value in your time spent together. And it is also to create more loving and fun memories together.

Don't get discouraged if they don't seem to respond as you would like at first. It may take a few tries. This way of being with them may feel a little strange in the beginning if you are not accustomed to doing these types of activities together. This may be a shift that they will have to get used to. In her later years, my mother dealt with depression and often wanted to share it with me, in fact at one point her conversations almost always turned negative. A dear counselor knew I loved my mother but no longer enjoyed her company because of these negative conversations. *She called it to my attention that I was letting Mom control our time together and that I needed to decide how I would like to spend time with my mom and "take charge" in creating what I could feel good about in relating to her.* The next time Mom started talking negatively with me when I went to see her I explained I did not enjoy that and I felt it was ruining our time together. I told her I would like to do some positive things with her but if she continued to be negative I would need to leave. I actually had to get up and leave twice, but from then on Mom let me take charge of our time together and it made a world of difference. I was able to encourage her back into being the sweet mom she had been most of my life.

So if you have a similar situation, don't give up. Don't become angry, be gentle but do take charge. Begin by creating positive moments, and in time they will join you or at the very least they will know you are doing your best and on some level that will mean something to them... Keep trying and give it some time.

On the other hand, some of your loved ones will jump at the opportunity to have fun and meaningful times with you. So... let's begin.....

Play music from our era for us often. Spend a little time online and order some of these if you don't have them.

Frank Sinatra
Dean Martin
The 40's, 50's and 60's
Elvis
Mitch Miller singalongs
Patti Page
Patsy Cline

(If you know some of them, sing along with them. The more interactive, the more you connect and relate.) Ask them their favorite singers. Music takes us back to a gentler time and provokes wonderful memories. I remember a gentleman, a retired engineer, who surprised me by asking if I knew *Do You Know the Muffin Man* and when I began to sing it tears rolled down his cheeks as he remembered his father singing that to him when he was a boy.

-Ask us about "our favorite things"

There is a sheet of questions for this in the back of this book

-Show us pictures of our favorite things

Photographs or pictures from old magazines or *Reminisce Magazine*, places, people, pets, flowers, travel – get ideas from the list

-Read us poetry

Perhaps good "classic" poetry from our era (You may fall in love with it yourself.) *I Must Go Down to The Sea Again*, or *If* or *Breathes there a man with soul so dead who never to himself has said, "This is my own, my native land…"* So many beautiful poems that can bring life to your loved ones. *One Hundred and One Famous Poems* is a great book.

-Share stories from the classics (Keep it light)

Little Women, Tom Sawyer, Wuthering Heights, Old Man & the Sea, there are endless lists on the internet or library. Reading a story together gives you something to look forward to each time you get together and you can laugh and cry and discuss – a great way to connect. Did you have a school teacher like I did in grade school who read a chapter of *Lassie* every day? She was my favorite teacher. Give Mom or Dad something to look forward to, a bit of a story hour every time you come.

-Read us short stories from the many *Chicken Soup for the Soul* series. Many of these take only a few minutes.

-Share things from *Reminisce Magazine* and leave copies for us.

-Rent movies that make us laugh. Lots of them. I know a lady who was completely crippled with arthritis – couldn't raise her arms above her waist – who rented and watched every funny movie she could find and within a month of watching them was able to lift her arms. Laughter is healing, scientifically so, and it's an obvious mood lifter that lingers with us and helps our memories together to be good ones.

-Dance with us. I have experienced men and women both lighting up to just a few steps of a waltz..... or a jitterbug

-Get us out in nature

If we are able to walk, keeping us walking and out in nature is the best way to revitalize us – but that is something we won't do alone as we get older. You may be very surprised at how much it will do for their spirits and yours.

-Take us on a picnic – let us get our feet in the grass or the water – then you might even massage them with some nice lotion or lavender oil.

This could be a full-scale picnic with a basket or cooler and great finger foods or just a snack or donut under a shady tree or by a river. It restores our soul.

-Find out places we would like to go and give us an experience of it with music, song, pictures, stories (This can be endless as you go to different cultures with us)

The example I gave you of Italy is just one. Be creative and intertwine your interests and theirs. If you like drumming, take them to Africa and bring your drum. If you like Paris, take them there with food and wine and pictures and music. There is NO end to this one and every adventure together can be fantastic!

Engage them in these activities. Ask them what they would like to do while in Venice, Italy. Let them picture a gondolier singing to them while they float through the waterways of Venice. Ask them their favorite movies of Italy, favorite actors, favorite songs. Take out Italy and put any other location in the world but travel together and make it fun!

-Take us to some entertainment. They might love an opportunity to put on something nice and go to a concert, play or symphony. Or dress casual and go to a concert in the park or an art fair. Be aware of any physical limitations they have but don't just assume they can't do it – ask.

-Watch old movies with them. Find out which actors or actresses they like and rent a movie or order one on Netflix. It is wonderful to watch some of those old movies but it makes us feel lonely when we can only watch them by ourselves. Pop some corn or grab our favorite treat for a night at the movies at home.

-If your loved one has a favorite sport, plan to watch with them along with popcorn or pretzels and a beer or soda. Dad would sure enjoy doing that with you and not alone. Invite him to your place to watch a game with you and the kids or friends.

-Give us a makeover. Many older women love a facial. You can give us one or take us to a nice store where there are pros to do it and plan to buy a couple of items we like.

-Buy us a sunny new dress, nightgown or robe. We women never outgrow our love of something pretty, or even better, something that makes us feel pretty. Dad might like a nice robe if he is in a retirement home or living with a family member.

-Bring us flowers. They don't have to be expensive floral arrangements. A bouquet from a store or some flowers from your yard, keeping us with some fresh flowers really lifts our spirits – perhaps even reminds us girls of when we were being courted.

-Take us home for a home-cooked meal. If at all possible get us into a home environment as often as you can. If it is not possible for you to provide us with living quarters with you or a family member, bring us to your house on some kind of a regular basis. You can sometimes also let us make something for you in our place or buy some of our favorite food and bring it over and share it with us. *Every memory made in*

41

the place we are living creates an energy that remains long after you have gone home.

-Bring us our favorite food or drink. A cookie from our favorite bakery, a pizza to share. Something you know we like and seldom have an opportunity to get.

-Take us out for a Pina Colada. Some of the best laughs I had with my mother after my dad passed away was when we would go to our favorite little Mexican restaurant and order a Pina Colada. Mom almost never drank alcohol so we would usually order a virgin colada or daiquiri but we took our time together and visited and laughed together and had our own "happy hour".

-Take us to a pet shop. It has been proven time and again, and even scientifically, the comforting or some-times "awakening" effect animals have on the elderly. If you have a pet bring it or take them where there are animals.

-Just sit and talk with us and be sure when you do to ask us questions so we can talk. I can't say often enough that if you ask us questions and become a good listener it brings us alive to share our stories and can bring up things that you didn't know about us. *Asking us questions makes us feel special.*

-Get us around babies and animals. My mother didn't know who I was for the last 3 years of her life and she seldom spoke, but when my daughter brought her baby to see his great grandma for the first time Mom reached for little Nathan and when he began to cry, much to our amazement, she rocked him in her arms, patted his little bottom and said, "There, there, sweetheart, don't cry." As she planted a gentle kiss on his cheek I sat there in amazement and tears slipped down my cheeks as Mom hadn't spoken a word in over a year. Babies and animals sometimes bring back natural instincts and can give them a moment you won't forget.

-Take us to the park. A simple thing but something you can enjoy together. Nature, like animals and babies can "wake up" something inside us, and it's also very healing.

-Take us on family outings or vacations. We love to be included – and just being invited means a great deal to us. Give some thought to some plans in which you could include us.

-Let us help "peel the potatoes" – bake the pie. Any possibility of helping lets us feel useful and lifts our spirits.

-Send us a card with some rose petals in it or a pressed flower. You might remember the words to the old song, *Little Things Mean A lot*. Sometimes you may think it will take you a lot of time to do something that lifts our spirits but it often only takes a moment to drop us a pretty card or even just an envelope with a with some rose petals or a colored leaf and an "I love you" note. If your loved one texts or emails take just a moment to say, "Thinking of you." I was having a particularly down day recently when I heard a ping on my cell phone and much to my delight I received a text and some photos from my sweet daughter-in-law. She and my son were vacationing in Switzerland. The pictures were beautiful. The text simply said, "We are thinking of you". It brightened my day so much to know with them all that far away in such a beautiful place they were thinking of me. It warmed my heart and lifted my mood immediately.

-Share as many good memories that you have had with us through the years as you can. You may from time to time share memories you have of your childhood or youth with a friend, a spouse or your children and that's great but *no one* would appreciate it more than that loved one who may be alone now. We would love to hear your fond memories of times we spent together. And…let them share their memories with you as well. The last time I was with my Aunt Gladys before she passed away she recounted stories she had shared with me many times and she finished by saying, "I know I've told you these things before, but when you get older the only thing you have are your memories." *When they tell their stories they relive their memories and it brings up emotions and even physical chemicals within their bodies that lift their spirits and rejuvenate them.* It's medicine, and all you have to do is listen and enjoy.

Let me share a few extra thoughts on this point. If memories are all we have left as we near the end of life how about creating as many good memories as we can??!! Now! When our loved ones, and in the future, ourselves, can't be as physically active to go and do as we once did. It is wonderful to be able to recall sweet, fun, laughable, lovable, moments from our past.

And, you can continue to create those moments now by using some of the ideas here.

-Let us know anything you've learned from us. *All of us want to know our life has made a difference and nothing is more important than knowing we have made a positive difference in the lives of those we love.* Don't let those words go unspoken when they mean so much.

-Compliment anything you find pleasing about us. The older we get the fewer compliments we get about our looks or accomplishments, so pour them on gener-ously – but only if they are genuine. I'm guessing you can find many things to compliment if you know how much it means to us. That reminds me of a very sweet moment I had with my mother just a few months before she passed. I went to see her but she was sleeping. I thought about just slipping away since I didn't want to wake her but then the thought came of slipping in bed behind her and spooning with her as she used to do with me when I was little. When I did she awoke and began just touching my arm and then looked back over her shoulder at me and smiled. And out came the last whole phrase she ever said to me. I said to her, "You are still beautiful, Mom." I saw a faint twinkle in her eye as she smiled and said, "Who are you trying to kid, kiddo?" And we both laughed as I held her. She hadn't spoken a sentence in more than a year until that moment and it would be the last one we shared. What a lovely moment to carry with me.

-Ask for our opinion. *Do you suppose you will ever get tired of knowing your opinions matter?* I haven't met anyone who wants to feel unimportant and many, and I do mean many or most, elderly people feel their opinions don't matter to others. It empowers us to know they still do, so ask our opinion whenever possible.

-Let us tell our stories even if they are repeats – I promise you the day will come when you would give anything to sit with us and hear our stories one more time. I hit on that one earlier but can't repeat enough how important it is for you to not just "let" us tell our stories but "invite" us to. Almost my entire relationship with my grandfather came from me asking him each time I came to…. "Tell me a story, Grandpa." Oh how he loved that, and how many laughs we had together.

-Help us create new memories with you by doing some of the above. Take pictures when we are together and upload them online and make little memory books for us to keep on our coffee table to look at when you aren't there.

-Never miss a chance to send us a card with some of the things you think and feel We will keep them close at hand and read them 'til they are tattered.

-Take us out for tea or have a lovely tea party with us at your place or ours. Take Dad to his favorite coffee shop – maybe he will see someone he knows and if he does, encourage a conversation time with an old friend.

KNOW that the more we see of you and our grand-children the longer and happier we will live.

-Create a wall of pictures for us. So we can remember and feel proud to show to others the history of our lives and loved ones in pictures.

-Take us to a senior's dance. Let us feel handsome or pretty again and watch the lights come on. Let us feel proud to have you as our escort.

-The last thing I will suggest is to take the time to get to know a few of our meaningful friends. It means so much for you to know them and for us to be able to introduce them to you. Perhaps plan a time when you will come to see us especially for that purpose – and if we are not up to preparing some refreshments, bring some with you. What a treat! What a delight!

And always remember, your touch absolutely feeds energy into our body, mind, and heart. Holding our hand, giving us a hug, holding us a moment or two melts us into a state of peace and assures us of your love and lingers long after you are gone.

I hope this is triggering ideas for you and I would love it if you would share your ideas with me and let me know some of your experiences. I can be contacted by email at LivingtheSeasonsofLife@gmail.com. You can also watch for when my website comes up in early 2018 which will be www.LivingtheSeasonsofLife.com

In Conclusion:

I realize if you are reading this book it is because you may be at a difficult place in life, making hard decisions. You are trying to make the best decisions you can and I admire and congratulate you on taking the time to consider your situation both from your own standpoint and from that of your loved ones. *I can honestly tell you that realizing and using the information in this little book can transform your experience and relationships.* I personally learned a great deal of what I share with you from my situation with my own mother as I came to understand a great deal about her wants and needs. It pains me to say I didn't understand as much as I could have about her fears nor did I have in my mind, or have on hand, an arsenal of all the suggestions I have made for you here. When I started making presentations in retirement and nursing homes and seeing the response of these dear souls, that is when I learned so much more about creating happiness with the elderly.

While I do have wonderful loving memories with my mother and aunt, it pains me that I did not know while my own mother was living how much better I could have made her life. I hope I can save you that pain and I hope you will see the lights come on in the eyes of your own loved ones, hear their stories, dance with them, sing with them and create and share beautiful memories. When that happens *it is amazing and fulfilling*. I hope my mom is listening and smiling down from heaven that I "got it" and can now help so many others. I pray this will bless you and yours richly and I would love to hear from you and hear your stories. Perhaps in a future book what you are doing now will help others if you care to share your stories with me. I hope to hear from many of you so email me at livingtheseasonsoflife@gmail.com.

Now, go ahead, have those conversations, and listen, deeply listen. Then go and begin creating beautiful memories together! I hope you'll tell me about them but most of all have fun with them. Share your love in your own special way. I can feel joy for you and your loved ones just imagining the difference this will make. If you get stuck and need some help, email me or leave a message on my website and I'll help if I can.

Love and blessings,
Marilyn

ADDENDUM

Suggestions:

*Start a library of music for your times together

    Mitch Miller singalongs
    Dean Martin
    Johnny Mathis
    Elvis
    Tennessee Ernie Ford
    Lawrence Welk
    Hits from the 40's, 50's, and 60's
    Ask for their favorites

*Collect pictures from magazines – be sure and get some with bright colors

    Pics from their era
    Animals, butterflies, pets
    Birds and Blooms magazine is a great source for colorful pictures.
    Pictures from *Reminisce Magazine* will take them back to happier times.

*Create the atmosphere that will "jiggle their brain cells"
  Aprons
  Pretty hankies
  Perhaps a perfume they love
  Hats
  A pretty tea set or teapot if they have a kitchen area

*Get books in large print

*Coloring books and colored pencils, pens, or crayons (perhaps by them a pretty boxed art set)

*Be sure they have a large print address book with phone numbers.

*Give them a pretty guest book where you and others can sign in each time you come so we can look back and remember and you will know when they have had other guests.

*Keep some of the various *Chicken Soup for the Soul* books around.

Guideposts comes in large print

*Put up a cork board and change the pictures from time to time

*Be sure they have a pretty calendar on the wall someplace and write dates on it for when you will be coming etc.

NOTES

About the Author

M ARILYN IS A MOTHER OF 4 ADULT CHILdren and 11 grandchildren.

She has 46 years' experience in various forms of life coaching, seminars, public speaking, natural health and healing, corporate training, sales training, couples workshops, and process communication, certified under behavioral scientist, Dr. Taibi Kahler. Marilyn has authored and taught seminars in the US, Canada, and Mexico.

She has a passion for helping people find and use their talents and has expertise in both inspiring and giving practical ways to develop potential in ourselves and others. She does that in this book for seniors and is working on a follow-up book to help people of all ages use their talents and give their gifts to the world. To follow more about this and her next book go to www.LivingInYourOwnTruth.com

Marilyn has a deep love and concern for the elderly and has held many programs in retirement homes helping the seniors remember, revitalize, and express their memories, talents and inner beauty. This, coupled with her own personal journey with her loved ones, has prompted the writing of this book in the hope of sharing with others some things that have made a significant and loving difference for her and those seniors whose lives she has touched.

At this time Marilyn does a small amount of personal coaching by phone. If you are interested go to her website and email her at

www.LivingtheSeasonsofLife.com .

A few more things to help you create those magic moments....

For My Favorite Things:

My Favorite Things: Lyrics

Raindrops on roses and whiskers on kittens
Bright copper kettles and warm
woolen mittens
Brown paper packages tied up with strings
These are a few of my favorite things
Cream colored ponies and crisp apple strudels
Doorbells and sleigh bells and schnitzel
with noodles
Wild geese that fly with the moon on
their wings
These are a few of my favorite things

Girls in white dresses with blue satin sashes
Snowflakes that stay on my nose
and eyelashes
Silver white winters that melt into springs
These are a few of my favorite things

When the dog bites
When the bee stings
When I'm feeling sad
I simply remember my favorite things
And then I don't feel so bad

Favorite Things List of Questions:
Name_____
Date:_____
Your favorite……..
Color
Season of the Year
Book
Poems
Places
Holiday
Songs
Author
Dress
Memory
Favorite Age
Teacher
Relatives
Candy
Pie
Foods
Movies
President
Year
Cartoon Character
Actor
Actress
Singers
City
Animal
Pet
Hobby
Do for fun or enjoyment
Place to relax – now …. or when you were young
Vacation

Christmas Songs, including kids Christmas

Rudolph the Red Nosed Reindeer: Lyrics

Rudolph, the red-nosed reindeer
had a very shiny nose.
And if you ever saw him,
you would even say it glows.

All of the other reindeer
used to laugh and call him names.
They never let poor Rudolph
join in any reindeer games.

Then one foggy Christmas Eve
Santa came to say:
"Rudolph with your nose so bright,
won't you guide my sleigh tonight?"

Then all the reindeer loved him
as they shouted out with glee,
Rudolph the red-nosed reindeer,
you'll go down in history!

All I Want for Christmas: Lyrics

All I want for Chrithmath
is my two front teef,
my two front teef,
see my two front teef
Gee, if I could only
have my two front teef,
then I could with you
"Merry Chrithmath."

It seems so long since I could say,
"Thister Thusie thitting on a thistle!"
Gosh oh gee, how happy I'd be,
if I could only whithle (thhhh, thhhh)

All I want for Chrithmath
is my two front teef,
my two front teef,
thee my two front teef.

Gee, if I could only
have my two front teef,
then I could with you
Merry Chrithmath!... Chrithmath

I'm Getting Nuttin' for Christmas: Lyrics

I broke my bat on Johnny's head;
Somebody snitched on me.
I hid a frog in sister's bed;
Somebody snitched on me.

spilled some ink on Mommy's rug;
I made Tommy eat a bug;
Bought some gum with a penny slug;
Somebody snitched on me.

Oh, I'm gettin' nuttin' for Christmas
Mommy and Daddy are mad.
I'm gettin' nuttin' for Christmas
'Cause I ain't been nuttin' but bad.

I put a tack on teacher's chair;
Somebody snitched on me.
tied a knot in Suzy's hair;
Somebody snitched on me.
did a dance on Mommy's plant.
Climbed a tree and tore my pants.
Filled that sugar bowl with ants;
Somebody snitched on me.

Oh, I'm gettin' nuttin' for Christmas
Mommy and Daddy are mad.
I'm gettin' nuttin' for Christmas
'Cause I ain't been nuttin' but bad.

So you better be good whatever you do
'Cause if you're bad, I'm warning you,
You'll get nuttin' for Christmas.

Silent Night

Silent night, holy night!
All is calm, all is bright.
Round yon Virgin, Mother and Child.
Holy infant so tender and mild,
Sleep in heavenly peace,
Sleep in heavenly peace

Silent night, holy night!
Shepherds quake at the sight.
Glories stream from heaven afar
Heavenly hosts sing Alleluia,
Christ the Savior is born!
Christ the Savior is born

Silent night, holy night!
Son of God love's pure light.
Radiant beams from Thy holy face
With dawn of redeeming grace,
Jesus Lord, at Thy birth
Jesus Lord, at Thy birth

White Christmas: Lyrics

I'm dreaming of a white Christmas
Just like the ones I used to know
Where the treetops glisten and children listen
To hear sleigh bells in the snow

I'm dreaming of a white Christmas
With every Christmas card I write
May your days be merry and bright
And may all your Christmases be white

I'm dreaming of a white Christmas
Just like the ones I used to know
Where the treetops glisten and children listen
To hear sleigh bells in the snow

I'm dreaming of a white Christmas
With every Christmas card I write
May your days be merry and bright
And may all your Christmases be white

Songwriters: Irving Berlin
White Christmas lyrics © Tratore

CPSIA information can be obtained
at www.ICGtesting.com
Printed in the USA
LVOW10s0736250118
563972LV00001B/40/P